Department of Health
Department for Education and Employment
Home Office

3/97

The Removal, Retention and use of Human Organs and Tissue from Post-mortem Examination

Advice from the Chief Medical Officer

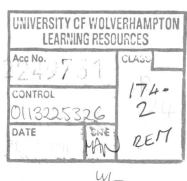

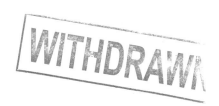

London

The Stationery Office

Contents

1 Introduction

This chapter sets out the background to, and purpose of, the report. It describes the sources of evidence, the views and the advice which have been drawn upon to formulate recommendations to the Government.

1   During the inquiry into the management of the care of children receiving complex heart surgery at Bristol Royal Infirmary, it emerged that the retention of hearts removed during post-mortem examination of the child's body had been commonplace. In many cases it appears to have taken place without parental consent or indeed knowledge.

2   Specifically, it emerged that a more extreme situation existed at Alder Hey Children's Hospital in Liverpool. The Alder Hey Inquiry has found that collections of children's hearts and other organs had been accumulated over several decades, in some cases as long as 50 years. The Inquiry established that it had been common practice to retain organs without express parental knowledge and agreement. Separate research collections held by the University of Liverpool included children's eyes, cerebella (part of the brain), body parts and fetuses.

3   The Alder Hey Inquiry also discovered that between 1988 and 1995 the then Professor of Fetal and Infant Pathology was responsible for the removal of all organs from all babies and children at post-mortem and their storage for intended research again apparently without parental knowledge or agreement. It appears that in the majority of cases, the organs were never put to any useful research purpose. In many cases, a proper post-mortem examination was never carried out and final reports on post-mortems were not produced.

4   Individuals and groups of relatives in other parts of the country have also made enquiries of local hospitals. The responses suggested the presence of substantial stores of retained human organs. This has been confirmed by the census, carried out during 2000, of organs and tissues retained by pathology services in England.

5   All these events have led to a great deal of public concern about past practice by pathology services in relation to the circumstances in which organs and tissues removed at post-mortem examination were kept over the long term for teaching or research. Those relatives directly involved, particularly in Bristol, Liverpool and Birmingham, have expressed deep distress, grief and anger over the discovery that their children's organs had been taken and kept without their knowledge. Their distress has been made worse by the way in which communications with them were managed following the revelations about the retained organs.

"Our main concern was the way the hospital dealt with our problems, being pushed from phone line to phone line, causing more distress and trauma for parents, being given information which was incorrect, leading to second burials, some parents refusing to bury until everything was clarified. Drip fed information: unless you asked the right questions you did not get the answers you wanted."

Lynne Langley
Stolen Hearts Group
Speaking at the CMO's Summit on 11th January 2001

6   During the controversy of the last few years, professional bodies and research charities have repeatedly drawn attention to the value of post-mortem examination and long-term study of retained organs and tissue in the advancement of medical science. Pathologists have stressed that practice was motivated by trying to do good for patients and never intended to cause distress or harm to families.

7   Few people, even the relatives caught up in these events, deny the benefits to patients that can flow from properly conducted research and from teaching using human organs and tissues: discovering the causes and effects of disease, establishing that some genetic diseases will affect other family members, even finding the cure for some fatal or disabling illnesses.

8   But something went seriously wrong in some institutions in the way that the health service and the medical profession sought to secure these advances in medical science and standards of care. Despite the fact that there is legislation governing the conduct of post-mortems and the retention of tissues and organs, there appears to have been little understanding or application of the law. It is also clear that assumptions were made about how families, particularly parents, felt about their loved ones after death. Some of this practice, at best, can be described as paternalistic and belonging to an era when decisions were made for patients and not with them.

"When a child died that child is still the parents' child – not a specimen, not a cause, not an unfortunate casualty of a failed procedure, but someone's baby, someone's child. In life the parent is responsible for every aspect of a child's well-being. In death that responsibility should not be taken away."

Stephen Parker
Bristol Heart Children's Action Group
Speaking at the CMO's Summit on 11th January 2001

9   In the last few years, changes have been introduced in many hospitals including more explicit consent forms for hospital post-mortem examination. These include explanations as to the difference between hospital post-mortems and coroners' post-mortems, more information for relatives on the purpose of the examination, more detailed descriptions of which organs and tissues are to be retained, and the reasons for requesting that organs and tissues should be retained beyond the time that the rest of the body is buried or cremated. These trends have been reinforced by interim guidance which I issued to the National Health Service in the Spring of 2000 and by guidelines which the Royal College of Pathologists issued at the same time.

"We feel most strongly that measures should be put into place so that what has been done to our children should never be allowed to happen again. Guidelines are not enough. It has been proven that they have been ignored. Self-regulation by the medical profession has been shown to be inadequate. We must have changes in the law that will cover both hospital and coroners' post mortems with clear concise rules and directives that are enforceable in law and that are designed to ensure that what happened to our children cannot be repeated in the future."

John O'Hare
PITY II Group, Liverpool
Speaking at the CMO's Summit on 11th January 2001

10   These measures are, however, not enough to address and put right the depth of the problem that has been uncovered. A new system must be introduced that is comprehensive and coherent, that addresses the important concerns raised by recent events, that draws in the views and experience of the families and their representatives and which takes on board the lessons of the two major inquiries – in Bristol and Alder Hey.

11   This is the task and the challenge addressed in this report to the Government.

12   In preparing my report I have drawn on:

- the interim report of the Bristol Royal Infirmary Inquiry (available at www.bristol-inquiry.org.uk).

- the report of the Royal Liverpool Children's NHS Trust (Alder Hey) Inquiry (available at www.rlcinquiry.org.uk/index.htm).

- the Summit Meeting on Organ Retention held in London on 11th January 2001 (proceedings and evidence available at www.cmosummit.org.uk).

- a wide range of written material, including current guidance from professional and research bodies, the Coroners' Society and submissions from members of the public.

- a series of meetings with representative groups and individuals both from the public, the professions and the health service. The organisations concerned are listed at Annex A.

- the census conducted in 2000 of organs and tissues retained by NHS pathology services in England at the end of 1999 (available at www.doh.gov.uk/organcensus).

13   I have not attempted to replicate the excellent analysis of the law found in the Interim Report of the Inquiry into the management of care of children receiving complex heart surgery at the Bristol Royal Infirmary, *Removal and Retention of Human Material* or that in the Report of the Royal Liverpool Children's NHS Trust Inquiry.

14   The intention is to provide definitive advice which will enable a new beginning and start the process of restoring public confidence. While much of the public attention has been on the taking and retention of organs from post-mortems on children, the report and the recommendations address post-mortem practice in all age groups.

Aims of the report

- to summarise the nature and scope of current and past practice in relation to the retention of organs and tissues;

- to draw together the main problems and concerns which have arisen from the operation of the system to date;

- to recommend comprehensive changes to current practice which will ensure:

  - a proper respect for the person who has died and the surviving relatives;

  - the compassionate treatment of bereaved families;

  - the provision of clear information and full explanations by clinicians on the purposes of organ and tissue removal and retention;

  - effective participation by families in taking key decisions so that any agreement to such procedures is freely given;

  - that, with the support of the public, the benefits of greater understanding of disease through research, audit and teaching, using retained tissue and organs after death, will help future generations of patients.

15   In considering the need for changes to address the serious problems and concerns about the practice of post-mortem examination, other related issues have become apparent. It is necessary to take stock comprehensively of the inter-relationship between the Human Tissue Act 1961, the Coroners' system and the process of death and cremation certification, and to consider weaknesses across the spectrum of law and guidance that impact in this area. Questions have also arisen about the importation of human material for teaching purposes, the commercial use of tissue and the controls on taking, using and storing tissue and organs removed from the living both for therapeutic or research purposes.

16   It was beyond the scope of this report to deal with all those wider matters. However, particular areas have been highlighted which will require further detailed consideration to identify workable solutions.

2

Removal, retention, use and disposal of organs and tissue after death: legal and regulatory issues

The removal of organs and tissues from the body after death for medical study can be undertaken for a number of purposes. The immediate tests and examinations carried out are to establish the cause of death. In some cases, organs and tissues are retained in pathology departments beyond the time of burial or cremation of the rest of the body and used for example in teaching or research. In this chapter, the legal and regulatory basis of this practice is described.

1   The examination of tissue and organs taken from the body is essential:

   - to establish the precise cause of death;
   - to diagnose the fatal disease accurately;
   - to identify the presence of unsuspected complications or other diseases;
   - to find out if death was related to an industrial disease, chemicals or poisons;
   - to ensure that lessons can be learned and more effective treatment given to future patients with the same disease.

2   In life, samples of tissue, taken through biopsy or other means, can enable for example: breast, cervical or bowel cancer to be detected in its early stages when there may be the chance of a cure; a potentially life-threatening infection to be treated; a baby's life to be saved in the womb; or a breakthrough to be achieved in understanding what causes a particular disease.

3   With greater understanding of genetics and the human genome, it is now becoming possible to map a person's genes and identify their susceptibility to certain diseases. It is only by building up such genetic maps from diseased and normal organs and tissue that it will be possible to identify the genes which mark someone out as at a higher risk of disease. While much of this work can be undertaken on newly donated tissue, it is also now possible to go back to stored samples. This creates the opportunity for new analyses and medical discoveries which were never foreseen when the tissue was originally taken.

4   Samples of tissue are taken from a living person only with their agreement either as part of their medical care or if they are participating in a research study. For young children, tissue can only be removed with agreement from a person with parental responsibility. For adults who are not capable of providing consent, tissue can only be taken in the best interests of the patient, for example to assist in diagnosis of their illness. Today, agreement is expected to be obtained by informed consent, in which people are given the information they need to be able to reach a balanced judgement based on sufficient understanding of what is involved (including risks as well as benefits).

5   Many of the benefits of the medical examination of tissue can be captured by studying tissue taken after death, as well as that taken in life. For example, genetic and other abnormalities which may affect surviving relatives can be identified; parents can be advised of the possibility of abnormalities affecting future children; and diagnosis and treatments for other patients can be improved. There have been many occasions in the past where the study of tissue after death had led to discoveries in medical science which have resulted in the saving of lives and the relief of suffering. This has particularly been so in the field of cancer research.

6   Maintaining and improving standards of care also depends upon learning, after death, whether the patient's diagnosis had been accurate, why the disease killed as and when it did, and whether treatment could have been improved. In some cases, it may mean that the life of the next patient to undergo the same treatment could be saved.

7   Some of the research studies using organs or tissues obtained after death are of major significance for the health of people in this country, for example:

- the analysis of organs following death to understand better the long-term effects of drug therapy, both to develop improved treatments and identify side-effects that might have gone unrecognised in life;

- the study of cells taken from organs after death to explore the way in which cancers progress or might be stopped from developing;

- the examination of tissue from people with Parkinson's Disease to understand the cause of this disease and potential cures, treatment and prevention;

- to study and monitor the levels of chemicals and radioactive elements absorbed from the environment.

8   There are also many examples where researchers have been able to go back to tissue collected many years previously and held in archives to establish important links in the causation of disease, for example, the study of brains of people who have died from dementia to investigate whether they have Alzheimer's disease or whether they are undiagnosed cases of variant Creutzfeldt-Jakob disease (vCJD).

9   Without the donation of tissue in life or after death it will not be possible in the future to realise the benefits of genetic research which has already yielded breakthroughs for example in the fields of breast and colon cancer from testing tissue held in archives.

10   Large-scale storage of human biological materials occurs in other countries. The 1999 report of the National Bioethics Advisory Commission (NBAC) in the United States of America (http://bioethics.gov/pubs.html) estimates that over 282 million specimens were stored and were accumulating at around 20 million specimens per year. This comprised all types of human biological material including blood, tissue samples taken during diagnosis or treatment as well as material taken after death. Individual collections of human biological materials ranged from fewer than 200 to more than 92 million individual quantities of material. They ranged from large tissue banks, repositories and organ banks to unique tissue collections covering specialist areas. The NBAC report does not identify the size of pathology holdings of organs or tissue specifically gathered after post-mortem examination but these are likely to be very substantial. The National Disease Research Institute provides 140 different types of human tissues obtained from post-mortem examination and delivers to researchers across the United States for research into over 100 different types of disease. Other repositories

in the United States loan pathological material for patient treatment or research, whilst banks of organs (e.g. brain banks) are also seen as a valuable resource for biomedical research or educational purposes.

11   Despite the benefits outlined, the use of organs and tissues after death (other than for transplantation) has become a source of serious public concern in this country. The taking and use of tissue during life has not appeared to raise the same level of concern.

12   Some tests carried out after death require laboratory preparation of the organ or tissue so that a proper examination can be made. This particularly applies to the brain. If brain disease or injury is suspected, it can only be properly diagnosed if the brain is 'fixed' with chemicals so that it can be examined by eye and under the microscope. The process of fixation takes about four weeks to complete, or may take longer. Thus, if the brain is being examined to establish the cause of death, in many cases burial or cremation of the body will already have happened. This raises the question of the subsequent disposal of the organ or tissue.

13   The reasons for concern about the removal and retention of tissues and organs after death (highlighted in Bristol and Alder Hey) appear to be:

  ● there has been no adequate recognition or acknowledgement, on the part of the majority of NHS staff or many doctors, of the feelings people have on the recent loss of a family member, particularly a child, and the extent to which they feel the need to protect a child even after that child's life ends;

  "The bond between the parent and child will not diminish because the child has died."

  Jenny Thomas
  Child Bereavement Trust
  Speaking at the CMO's Summit on 11th January 2001

  ● the majority of post-mortem examinations are carried out as part of the legal process for establishing the cause of death, under the auspices of the coroner and are compulsory – relatives have no say or choice in the matter;

  "I would suggest that it was precisely because people were working in isolation and not communicating properly and not listening to one another that we are in the situation in which we find ourselves today. It is a situation that has taken its toll on many people and on many processes: on the families and next of kin traumatised by these events, who have had old wounds reopened and old griefs reawakened, and who feel mistreated and betrayed by a system in which they built an absolute trust."

  Niall Weir
  Hospital Chaplaincies' Council
  Speaking at the CMO's Summit on 11th January 2001

- in the past, the level of information given, the skill in supporting bereaved people and the standard of communication with relatives have all been relatively poor in the NHS;

- the law in this area is old-fashioned, ambiguous and tilted towards marginalising families rather than ensuring that they are equal partners in the decision-making process. In any event there has been a lack of understanding of the law and it has sometimes been ignored.

Two main types of examination after death

14   Organs or tissues are taken from a person's body after death as part of one of two main processes: a coroner's post-mortem examination, carried out by a pathologist designated by the coroner, or a hospital post-mortem examination (sometimes called a 'consent' post-mortem) carried out by a pathologist working in a hospital. Each is governed by separate legislation.

Coroner's post-mortem

15   About a third of all deaths in England and Wales are reported to coroners. The coroner may then decide to order a post-mortem examination. An inquest may also be necessary. Approximately 62% of the deaths reported to the coroner undergo post-mortem examinations, but only 12% of reported deaths result in inquests. In the majority of cases the post-mortem examination is sufficient to determine the cause of death and an inquest is not required. The duties of coroners are governed by the Coroners Rules 1984 and the Coroners Act 1988. Specifically, the Coroners Rules govern the taking and retention of organs and tissues during the post-mortem process.

16   A post-mortem examination is requested by the coroner when the cause of death is uncertain and needs to be determined. This does not mean that all such deaths are thought to be suspicious or sinister. Circumstances in which a coroner's post-mortem would be ordered include sudden or unexpected deaths. Examples include the death of a child after surgery, the death of an adult who collapses for no apparent reason or any death where the person has not recently been seen by their general practitioner. The purpose of the coroner's post-mortem is limited in law to establishing that the cause of death was 'natural'.

17   The retention of tissue and organs is similarly limited to establishing the cause of death, although this appears to be ill-understood.

> *"A person making a post-mortem examination shall make provision, so far as possible, for the preservation of material which in his opinion bears upon the cause of death, for such period as the Coroner thinks fit".*
>
> (Coroners Rules 1984 – Rule 9)

18   There are a number of features of the coroner's post-mortem arrangements particularly relevant to the subject of this report.

Key features of the coroner's post-mortem system

- the decision to carry out the post-mortem is at the discretion of the coroner;

- the coroner chooses the pathologist;

- the relatives have no choice over whether the post-mortem goes ahead – it is in effect compulsory;

- in practice, much of the communication with the relatives and the pathologist are by the coroner's officer, not the coroner himself/herself;

- organs or tissue cannot be taken from the body for any purpose except to establish the cause of death; nor can they be retained longer than necessary to establish that sole purpose;

- the relatives are entitled to be represented at the post-mortem examination (e.g. by their general practitioner). Few are, as this is rarely practical in view of the need to hold the examination relatively quickly;

- the coroner's post-mortem examination is not carried out to an approved or standard pattern around the country, is not necessarily a full post-mortem of the kind necessary to audit the standard of care and is merely directed towards establishing whether the death was 'natural' or 'unnatural';

- after a coroner's post-mortem, the coroner completes the death certificate;

- a copy of the post-mortem examination report can be provided to the family for a fee;

- there is a lack of clarity on the rules for disposing of retained tissue once the necessary tests or inquest are completed.

Hospital post-mortem

19   Provided there is no objection from relatives, a hospital post-mortem examination can be carried out on a person who has died, in order to gain a fuller understanding of the deceased's illness or the cause of death so as to enhance future medical care. It can also be carried out to obtain 'tissue' or any part from the body for therapeutic purposes or for the purposes of future medical education or research. Strictly speaking, this kind of post-mortem is not a legally required examination to establish the cause of death, which is the purpose of a coroner's post-mortem. The authorisation for taking and retaining tissue and organs from the hospital post-mortem is governed by the Human Tissue Act 1961, which also governs taking tissue, such as corneas, for transplantation.

Extracts from Human Tissue Act 1961

1. Removal of parts of bodies for medical purposes

(1) If any person, either in writing at any time or orally in the presence of two or more witnesses during his last illness, has expressed a request that his body or any specified part of his body be used after his death for therapeutic purposes or for purposes of medical education or research, the person lawfully in possession of his body after his death may, unless he has reason to believe that the request was subsequently withdrawn, authorise the removal from the body of any part or, as the case may be, the specified part, for use in accordance with the request.

(2) Without prejudice to the foregoing subsection, the person lawfully in possession of the body of a deceased person may authorise the removal of any part from the body for use for the said purposes if, having made such reasonable enquiry as may be practicable, he has no reason to believe:

(a) That the deceased had expressed an objection to his body being so dealt with after his death and had not withdrawn it; or

(b) That the surviving spouse or any surviving relative of the deceased objects to the body being so dealt with.

20   There are a number of relevant features of the hospital post-mortem:

Key features of hospital post-mortem system

- The active consent of relatives is not needed: it must simply be established that the relatives (or the deceased) do not/did not object to such an examination. In practice most hospitals ask for a signature on a form;

- organs and tissue are not referred to or defined;

- there is no express requirement under the law to give particular information to relatives. In practical terms, establishing lack of objection requires discussion with relatives and the provision of basic information;

- there is no defined legal limit to the amount of 'tissue' that can be retained (ie there is no barrier to retaining whole organs or body parts);

- legally, the person 'in possession of the body' can be the hospital rather than the relatives and a member of the hospital staff can therefore authorise the removal of organs and tissue.

Guidance on post-mortem examination

21   Professional bodies issue guidance to their members from time to time on appropriate standards of practice for the removal and retention of tissue. Of particular relevance is guidance from the Royal College of Pathologists which includes:

- *Guidelines for Post-Mortem Reports.* Royal College of Pathologists 1993. These guidelines outline the standard that should be applicable to all post-mortem examinations including coroners' post-mortems. They also describe how the report should provide clear information for the clinician, coroner, general practitioner and the pathologist;

- *Guidelines for the Retention of Tissue and Organs at Post-Mortem Examination* issued in March 2000. These guidelines are intended to help all doctors, particularly pathologists, and coroners and their staff make decisions on the issue of retention of tissues and organs at post-mortem; and to ensure that the examination of the body after death continues to have public support and is conducted in a respectful manner in which the public has confidence. The guidance includes a plain English new 'model form' for agreement to post-mortem.

22   The Coroners' Society for England and Wales provides guidance for coroners: *Practice Notes for Coroners.* Coroners' Society of England and Wales 1998. The Coroners' Society's Notes remind coroners about the relevant statutory rules which apply where a post-mortem examination is ordered by a coroner, and offer views on good practice. This includes the need to avoid delay; to choose an appropriately qualified pathologist; to consider, when choosing the pathologist, whether any conflicts of interest arise; to provide the family of the deceased with appropriate information about the examination, if necessary in writing; and to keep the family advised of any delay and of the result of the examination. The Notes also stress the limitations of the scope of the examination, and the need to proceed in accordance with the provisions of the Human Tissue Act 1961 or the Anatomy Act 1984 if a wider examination or research is required.

23   In addition, in March 2000 the Department of Health issued *Interim Guidance on Post-Mortem Examination* which requires NHS Trusts to:

- ensure all staff who have contact with bereaved relatives have proper understanding of, and respect for, the rights of the dead;

- designate a named individual to provide support and information to families of the deceased where a post-mortem examination may be required;

- provide clear written information about the options for the disposal of organs, body parts and tissues retained at post-mortem, including arrangements for reuniting these with the body;

- ensure professional staff follow best practice;

- obtain 'consent' to post-mortem on a signed form and provide a copy to the relative who signed it;

- have proper systems in place for recording the details of all post-mortems including: whether consent was obtained; where organs, body parts or tissue were retained; and how retained organs and tissues were archived or disposed of;

- ensure the disposal is in accordance with wishes expressed by the deceased prior to death or by relatives.

Post-mortem examination of fetuses and stillborn children

24   When a fetus is born dead at or before 24 weeks gestation the law does not require the birth to be certified or registered. For babies stillborn after 24 weeks, the stillbirth must be certified on a special certificate. No legal provisions apply to the examination of fetuses or to the removal or retention of tissue. However, taking fetuses or fetal material for use in research or treatment does fall under the terms of the Code of Practice on the Use of Fetuses and Fetal Material in Research and Treatment drawn up in 1989 by the Polkinghorne Committee (the Polkinghorne Guidelines).

Key features of the Polkinghorne Guidelines

- there should be clear separation between decisions and actions relating to terminating the pregnancy and decisions and actions relating to the use of fetal material made available;

- the written consent of the mother should be obtained before any research involving the fetus or fetal tissue takes place;

- consent to the termination of pregnancy must be given before consent is sought to the use of fetal tissue;

- no inducements, financial or otherwise, should be put to the mother, or those who may influence her, to allow fetal tissue to be used;

- all proposals for the use of fetuses or fetal tissue must be referred to a research ethics committee in recognition of the sensitivity surrounding the use of such tissue.

Review of the Guidance on the Research Use of Fetuses and Fetal Material London HMSO July 1989.

25   Stillbirths are not reportable to the coroner. However, the coroner may become involved where it is necessary to determine whether the dead infant was truly stillborn or died from some other cause after birth.

26   Guidance to professionals is provided in: *The Fetal and Infant Post-Mortem: Brief Notes for the Professional.* (Confidential Enquiry into Stillbirths and Death in Infancy (CESDI) 1998). This recommends that consent for examination is obtained for all fetuses. A leaflet helps professionals answer parents' questions when a post-mortem is being considered. It provides advice on good practice and further information to assist those discussions that accompany a request for post-mortem. It also covers feedback to parents and information about the coroner's post-mortem, mainly relevant to post-mortems on infants.

Donations of bodies for anatomical examination

27   The Anatomy Act 1984 enables people, prior to their death, to bequeath their bodies for anatomical examination by dissection for teaching, studying or research purposes.

28   Each year, approximately 1,000 adults decide to bequeath their bodies for the benefit of medical education and science under the terms of the Anatomy Act. This Act enables medical, dental and other students in health related professions to learn about human anatomy and to undertake dissection so that they better understand human anatomy for the benefit of their subsequent professional careers. However, while the Anatomy Act allows dissection, it does not permit new surgical operative techniques to be performed or for any research to be undertaken that is not directly related to the study of anatomy.

29   Approximately 800 bodies per year are actually donated under the Anatomy Act and are usually bequeathed to the medical school nearest the person's home. A person bequeathing their body can also give permission for parts of their body to be retained permanently for teaching.

30   All medical schools receiving bodies bequeathed under the Anatomy Act are required to notify HM Inspector of Anatomy whenever a body is received; to retain the bequeathal form and other documentation for subsequent inspection and to notify HM Inspector of Anatomy when the body has been disposed of. All anatomy departments, which the Act requires to be licensed, are subject to regular inspections. HM Inspector of Anatomy makes an annual report to the Secretary of State. Thus bodies or body parts are subject to a strict control regime set out in the Anatomy Act and Regulations, and compliance is monitored through inspection by HM Inspector.

Key features of donations under the Anatomy Act 1984 and Anatomy Regulations 1988

- a request from an adult that his/her body should be used after death for anatomical examination, must be made in writing or exceptionally may be made orally in the presence of two witnesses during the person's final illness;

- the provision which allows authorisation by the person lawfully in possession of the body provided he/she has no reason to believe that the deceased or surviving relatives object has not been used in recent years, as the number of bodies bequeathed prior to death has been sufficient;

- a bequeathed body must be disposed of by burial or cremation within 3 years of death;

- body parts may be retained for separate study with the permission of the person bequeathing their body and the agreement of his/her relatives;

- body parts can only be used for anatomical examination, which includes dissection and visual examination;

- full records of bodies and all anatomical specimens, their use and disposal must be retained for at least 5 years;

- disposal must be in accordance with any expressed wishes of the deceased;

- HM Inspector of Anatomy inspects premises where bodies for anatomical examination and anatomical specimens are kept, their record keeping and disposal practices.

Other donations of bodies and body parts for medical science

31   Donations of whole bodies or body parts may also be made under the Human Tissue Act 1961. The Human Tissue Act 1961 does not contain the documentary requirements of the Anatomy Act and donations are not subject to review by HM Inspector of Anatomy. Donations made under the Human Tissue Act 1961 would permit the practice of new surgical operative techniques and non-anatomical research, which are excluded by the Anatomy Act. The Human Tissue Act 1961 does not include any requirements for disposal of body parts within a specific period. Thus, the Human Tissue Act 1961 contrasts with the strict control regime required under the Anatomy Act 1984 and Anatomy Act Regulations 1988.

Consent

32   There is no English statute setting out the general principles of consent to treatment. Case law ("common law") has established that, in the context of treatment, consent must be given by a competent person, acting voluntarily, who is informed in broad terms about the nature and purpose of the procedure. Parents can give such consent for their children under 18 years, although children over 16 years, and younger children with the necessary competence and understanding, can give their own consent.

33   The term "informed consent" has not historically been part of the English law on consent. Legally it tends to be used to refer to an "objective" standard used in some North American jurisdictions where the patient must be given the amount of information that "a reasonable person, in what the physician knows or should know to be the patient's position would be likely to attach significance to". This standard was rejected in a House of Lords case in 1985 (*Sidaway*).

34   In England, clinicians have only had to demonstrate that their practice (on provision of information) was in accordance with a responsible body of medical opinion. It has therefore primarily been profession-led rather than patient-led or to an objective standard.

35   However English law may be changing. A 1998 case in the Court of Appeal (*Pearce v. UBHT*) stated that it will normally be the responsibility of a doctor to inform a patient of "a significant risk which would affect the judgement of a reasonable patient". A patient's right to information is therefore starting to be recognised in law.

36   Professional practice is also changing with the most recent guidance from both the General Medical Council (GMC) and the British Medical Association (BMA) recognising the need for the relationship between doctor and patient to be based on the concept of partnership. The GMC's guidance – *Seeking Patients' Consent: The Ethical Considerations (1998)* – sets out the principles of good practice which all registered doctors are expected to follow when seeking patients' informed consent to investigation, screening or research. This includes giving patients sufficient information in order for them to exercise their right to make informed decisions about their care.

"Because we view consent as one of the foundations of good clinical practice and we believe that the test as to whether sufficient information has been given to enable consent to be expressed should be determined by what the patient wishes or needs to know rather than what the doctor believes to be sufficient."

Sir Cyril Chantler
General Medical Council
Speaking at the CMO's Summit on 11th January 2001

37   The BMA will shortly publish a 'Consent Took Kit' which will provide a prompt to doctors on the factors to be considered when they are seeking consent as a means of improving practice in this area. There is also evidence from a survey undertaken by the BMA in preparing the Tool Kit that medical schools are now placing considerable importance on teaching about consent and communications.

38   The Department of Health is currently reviewing how to improve consent practice through its Good Practice in Consent Initiative, involving professional bodies and patient groups.

39   The law and guidance in the field of consent applies to the living and not to the dead. While the provision of information is clearly a pre-requisite for valid consent to be given by or on behalf of a living person, the position for relatives after a person's death is far less certain. This has not been a major feature of discussions on consent up to now. The Human Tissue Act 1961 refers to "lack of objection" of a relative, and it is not clear the extent to which this needs to be an "informed" lack of objection. The Courts could only consider the issues on a case by case basis and are therefore unlikely to provide consistent and transparent standards that could apply to the provision of information before post-mortems, or taking and retaining organs after post-mortems.

"I think fundamentally there are two potentially and they need not be conflicting but they are potentially conflicting themes. The first which has been touched on by more than one speaker is to recognise that there is a value to research, to education and to patient care in being able to retain organs. But the second and the more important one is to recognise the central place of taking consent or, as we might wish in the BMA perhaps to use the term, asking permission from family members before examinations and the retention of organs can proceed and fundamentally that the consent must be fully informed."

Dr Michael Wilks
Chairman
British Medical Association's Ethics Committee
Speaking at the CMO's Summit on 11th January 2001

The Human Rights Act 1998

40   The Human Rights Act 1998 came into force in England on 2 October 2000 and incorporated the European Convention on Human Rights into domestic law. For public authorities (for example NHS Trusts), the Human Rights Act 1998 makes it a legal duty to act in accordance with the rights laid down in the Convention, unless any legislative provisions make it impossible for the authority to do so.

41   Where legislation is found to be incompatible with one of the Convention rights, a Court can make a 'declaration of incompatibility'. Where public authorities, such as NHS Trusts, do not act compatibly with the Convention rights, their actions will be 'unlawful' unless their actions related to compliance with current legislative provision. An individual will be able to take the public authority to Court if their rights under the Convention have not been observed.

42   The main Article of the Convention of potential relevance to removing, retaining and using tissue is Article 8.

Article 8: European Convention on Human Rights
"Everyone has the right to respect for his private and family life, his home and his correspondence".

43   It is possible that the lack of an effective sanction for wrongful removal of tissue – such as failure to comply with the Human Tissue Act 1961 by establishing "lack of objection" from relatives or retention without the opportunity for relatives to object or the use of retained tissue in ways which could affect a surviving relative's well-being (e.g. genetic research) – might all be considered incompatible with Article 8. However, the question of whether removal, retention and use of tissue from a dead family member constitutes lack of respect for private and family life has not been considered by the Courts.

The Council of Europe Convention on Human Rights and Biomedicine

44   This Convention of the Council of Europe is designed to protect the dignity and integrity of human beings and to guarantee respect for their rights and freedoms with regards to the application of biology and medicine.

45   A number of Articles of the Convention are relevant to the consideration of taking, storing and using tissue and organs.

Relevant Articles of the Convention on Human Rights and Biomedicine

Article 2

"The interest and welfare of the human being shall prevail over the sole interest of society or science".

Article 5

"An intervention in the health field may only be carried out after the person concerned has given free and informed consent to it.

This person shall beforehand be given appropriate information as to the purpose and nature of the intervention as well as on its consequences and risks.

The person concerned may freely withdraw consent at any time".

Article 22

"When in the course of an intervention any part of a human body is removed, it may be stored and used for a purpose other than that for which it was removed, only if this is done with appropriate information and consent procedures".

46   Although the Convention is concerned with the protection of living individuals, the principles laid down may also be relevant to taking and retaining organs at post-mortem.

Disposal of organs and tissue following post-mortem

47   The vast majority of tissues, organs and body parts, when no longer needed following laboratory investigation, for storage or for use in research or teaching are disposed of as clinical waste. This method is also used to dispose of tissues, organs and body parts removed during surgery.

> "When my son died 6 years ago all I received back for the first burial was his skull, his two arms, his two legs, hands, feet and about four ribs and his skin. Everything else was kept. When I received back my tissue box and samples they were so tiny what actually happened to the rest of the organ that they cut off? I was told it was respectfully cremated. I have further found out that it was thrown in a yellow waste bag as clinical waste and disposed with a disposal unit that empties dustbins. Now, can you tell me if that is respectfully cremated? Because nobody can tell me where these remains are now because it was put in an incinerator and they will be on a tip somewhere. Now, why are we still being lied to when we have had the worst possible thing that could happen to us again and you are still sat there lying to us?"
>
> Parent
> Speaking at the CMO's Summit on 11th January 2001

48   Safety in handling and disposal of clinical waste has been the primary consideration in guidance issued to the NHS over recent years, rather than the need for respectful disposal or consultation with the next of kin. A Strategic Guide to Clinical Waste Management for General Managers and Chief Executives was issued to the NHS in January 1994. Further guidance on the management of clinical waste, *Safe Disposal of Clinical Waste*, produced by the Health Services Advisory Committee was published in September 1999. All existing guidance recommends incineration for the disposal of human tissue. European Directives also cover safe disposal of human organs and tissues as waste but again say nothing about the wishes and intentions of relatives of the person who has died.

49   Regulations which came into force on 14 February 2000 (the Cremation (Amendment) Regulations 2000) allowed for organs or tissue removed and retained during the course of a post-mortem examination to be cremated where the body had previously been buried. This had not previously been permitted. This regulation does not apply to body parts retained from bodies donated under the Anatomy Act 1984.

> *"We have heard a lot today about how important medical research is to the progression of medical science and the value the profession places on the continued access to this valuable human material. Members of the profession have voiced concerns about the decline in the amount of post mortems being carried out, but what beggars belief is that this vast majority of the so-called valuable human material has been discarded as clinical waste in the past. The message sent out from this practice is that this human material was obviously not as valuable as the medical profession has had us or have led us to believe. Therefore, my question today is how can the public be convinced of the importance of this continued access to human material, when it is treated without respect or dignity, and is discarded with no more thought than society deals with its domestic rubbish?"*
>
> Parent
> Speaking at the CMO's Summit on 11th January 2001

50   Advice from the Home Office is that body parts taken from the body at post-mortem may be buried whether or not the body was buried. Although there is no specific provision for the separate burial of body parts, there is no legislation to prevent this.

51   There has been greater recognition of the need to consider the views of relatives when making arrangements for the disposal of fetuses and fetal material. Guidance is framed on the principle that the dead fetus should be shown respect based upon its lost potential for life and full human development. Since guidance was issued in 1991 (Disposal of Fetal Tissue HSG(91)19 and Sensitive disposal of the dead fetus and fetal tissue (EL(91)144)) NHS Trusts have been required to:

- take account of any wishes expressed by parents about disposal (choices might include burial, cremation, memorials, photographs and other mementoes.)
- store fetal tissue in separate, secure, opaque containers.

52   There is evidence from the 2000 census of organs and tissues retained by pathology services that recent practice has generally followed this guidance.

53   Fetuses over 24 weeks gestation may be cremated under the procedures set out in the cremation regulations for stillbirths. The subsequent cremation of tissue retained from stillbirths is not included in the Amendment Regulations referred to above and would not be permissible.

54   The Cremation Regulations do not apply to pre-viable fetuses (ie those under 24 weeks gestation) although cremation authorities have the discretion to permit their cremation. Tissue removed from fetuses of less than 24 weeks gestation may also be cremated at the cremation authority's discretion. There is therefore an inconsistency between what is permitted for tissue retained from stillbirths and for tissue from pre-viable fetuses.

Other legal considerations

55   A number of other areas of law in this field including rights to possession of a body and the ownership of body parts were helpfully reviewed in evidence given to the Bristol Inquiry and can be found on the Inquiry's web site (www.bristol-inquiry.org.uk).

3 Past and present practice: issues and concerns

The previous chapter described the law, as well as professional and NHS guidance governing the removal and retention of organs and tissues for medical examination or study after death. This chapter discusses the problems and concerns that have arisen in the operation of the system. The analysis of this situation draws on the key issues identified by the two inquiries (Alder Hey and Bristol), the census carried out in 2000 of pathology services in England, the views of families and of a wide range of organisations who presented evidence at the National Summit meeting.

1   Post-mortem examination is an essential element of the coroners' system in England, not just for the investigation of deaths where there are suspicious circumstances but for dealing with those which are sudden or unexpected or relate to industrial disease. Post-mortem examination has also played an important role in medical practice – in teaching and training doctors, in understanding disease, in auditing standards of care, and in finding new and better ways of treating patients.

2   The legislation governing the examination of the body after death and the retention and further medical use of organs and tissues taken after death is between 15 and 40 years old.

3   Within a framework of ageing legislation, which is in places unclear and ambiguous, some guidance has been produced over the years. However, in the last 30 years, the system has operated on a 'custom and practice' basis. It is the extent to which this has fallen out of step with public understanding and public expectations which is at the heart of the present controversy.

> *"Histopathologists, as well as parents, are also very distraught. They were always acting, they believed, in the interest of the families concerned and were trying to discover more about the precise cause of death and to learn more about the diseases involved."*
>
> *"That was in the past and we now fully realise and completely accept that this somewhat paternalistic approach may have been acceptable practice some years ago but is certainly not now."*
>
> Professor John Lilleyman
> President, Royal College of Pathologists
> Speaking at the CMO's Summit on 11th January 2001

Post-Mortem Rates

4   Statistics show that the overall post-mortem rate has shown a slight decline over the past three decades. In the early 1970s, approximately 28% of all deaths were followed by a post-mortem examination; with the percentage in 1999 being 25%. The proportion of post-mortems which are coroners' post-mortems has risen over that period. Of the 139,000 post-mortems carried out in 1999, approximately 90% (125,000) were coroners' post-mortems and 10% (14,000) were hospital post-mortems.

Table 1: Trend in post-mortems 1970–1999

Time period	Registered Deaths	Coroners' post-mortems	Hospital post-mortems
1970 – 1989	11,630,000	2,750,000	480,000
1990 – 1998	5,065,000	1,144,000	180,000
1999	553,000	125,000	14,000

Note: all figures rounded to the nearest 1,000.

5   The decline of the hospital post-mortem from the 1970s has been dramatic. It was once seen as an important element of hospital practice. Consultants, junior doctors and medical students would often attend post-mortems at the end of the morning ward round in order to discuss with the pathologist deaths under the care of that particular team. This was a valuable way of auditing the standard of practice, teaching students, training junior staff and learning more about disease. Under the terms of the Human Tissue Act 1961, the hospital post-mortem became the main route through which organs and tissue were retained over the long term for teaching and research purposes. The hospital post-mortem is today less common, possibly because doctors are less willing to ask relatives for permission and families may be less inclined to agree.

6   There has been a variable approach around the country in :

- the extent to which post-mortem examinations were sought and carried out;
- the nature and scale of retention and storage of organs, body parts and tissue beyond the time necessary for establishing the cause of death;
- the uses to which such retained material have been put;
- practice in obtaining consent.

7   As a consequence, at the end of 1999 NHS hospital and university medical schools had a total approximate holding of nearly 105,000 organs and body parts, stillbirths and fetuses. About half of these holdings have been accumulated over the last 30 years, whilst the remainder relate to pre-1970 (with some dating to the 19th century or earlier).

8   These numbers, derived from the census of organs and tissues held by pathology services in England carried out in 2000, are only estimates because standards of cataloguing and record keeping were not uniformly high. Therefore, definitive figures cannot be given and it is possible that the true numbers may be higher than those cited in the census report.

9   While many such retentions apparently took place after a hospital post-mortem under the Human Tissue Act 1961, there was evidence from the census that NHS Trusts had retained organs and tissues from coroners' post-mortems beyond the time necessary to establish the cause of death, for example:

- 16,000 organs and body parts obtained from coroners' post-mortems between 1970 and 1999 were retained in 85 NHS Trusts at the end of 1999.

- tissue samples were retained from one-third of coroners' post-mortems between 1970 and 1999, probably as a result of guidance that tissue blocks and slides should be retained as part of the medical record. The status of such blocks and slides is however unclear.

The basis of the past retentions

10   Taking account of what is known about past practice as demonstrated by the two inquiries and the census, it is difficult to be sure what the basis of a retention, of which relatives were not fully aware, actually was. Broadly, however, it seems to have fallen into one or more of the following categories:

- taking and retention was authorised through a hospital post-mortem after a family member had signed a form soon after the death but had been unaware what they were really signing for. While this may have complied with the letter of the Human Tissue Act 1961, it fell well short of any concept of informed consent or the spirit of the Act;

- taking and retention was authorised through a hospital post-mortem after a family member had been spoken to by a member of the hospital staff to ascertain whether they objected – again this may have technically complied with the Human Tissue Act 1961 but is equally short of being acceptable consent;

- taking and retention was authorised under the Human Tissue Act 1961 by a representative of the hospital who was "in possession of the body" who had satisfied themselves (however cursorily) that no-one 'objected'. Again this probably complies with the letter but goes against the spirit of consent (unless genuinely no living relative could be located after an extensive search);

- taking and retention was authorised under the Human Tissue Act 1961 by obtaining a signature at the time the family member was informed that a (compulsory) coroner's post-mortem was required. This may technically comply with the Act but does not appear appropriate, as it could lead someone to think they had no choice but to sign;

- taking and retention followed a coroner's post-mortem in the belief that there was a local understanding with coroners that this could be done for purposes such as teaching and research; it was general and accepted practice (though not within the law); and pathologists extended their usual retention practice to coroners' post-mortems; or there was a belief that, following post-mortem, families had lost any 'rights' to the tissues and organs. There would be no suggestion of attempting to obtain consent from families in this situation.

11   Anyone who reflects on past custom and practice for taking and retaining organs and tissue which had built up within an unclear and ageing framework of legislation would recognise that it had become significantly out of step with modern day expectations.

The Human Consequences

12   The end result of this system of authorising the removal and long-term retention of organs and tissues after the various types of post-mortem examination is that hospitals and medical schools were holding in storage extensive collections of human material of which relatives were largely unaware.

> *"We have all learned that our children's organs have been removed and retained at post mortem examination without our knowledge or consent. We are led to believe that this practice has been taking place since 1947. We have parents in our group who are revisiting the painful grief of 40, 30, 20 years ago and, indeed, as recently as 1999."*

> Mr John O'Hare
> Committee Member of PITY II Parents Support Group
> Speaking at the CMO's Summit on 11th January 2001

13   It is quite clear from the report of the two inquiries – Bristol and Alder Hey – that the parents of children whose organs and tissues were stored in pathology departments and academic institutions had believed that they had buried or cremated their child intact. When the fact of the retention of children's hearts, brains and other organs came to light, there was outrage, grief and distress which has continued unabated over a two year period.

14   The accounts of the experiences of the parents in Liverpool, Bristol and other cities, which were presented to the inquiries and given as testimony at the National Summit, are extremely harrowing accounts. They reveal more than a simple misunderstanding of the purpose and techniques of traditional medical practice. They reveal much more deep-seated problems.

> *"It almost was – I mean, if I could just use an analogy, it was almost like scrap cars being taken to a scrapyard. The cars were dismantled, the alternators were taken out, the batteries were taken out, put on a shelf, then when somebody comes along and wants one of those parts they pay for it. In the case of our children, they were dissembled completely. The organs were stored, never used."*

> Parent
> Speaking at the CMO's Summit on 11th January 2001

15   They show a failure by many doctors, not all, to empathise with parents who have faced the devastating loss of a child and the failure to recognise that a parent feels love and the need to protect a child, even after death. The fact that for many parents the essence of a child is contained in organs such as the heart or the brain, engendered feelings that the child had been violated and that the parent had not been able to protect him or her.

16   This was compounded by the fact that:

- some were explicitly told that the organs had been returned to the body before burial when in fact this was not true;

"Lessons should be learned so that when people find out that they are involved with organ retention they should be dealt with in an understanding, sensitive and compassionate manner and should receive prompt and truthful answers to the questions, which has not always been the case at Alder Hey."

John O'Hare
PITY II Group, Liverpool
Speaking at the CMO's Summit on 11th January 2001

- parents were often given inaccurate information about what was and was not being held and some initial information proved misleading;

- when organs were returned this was often done in an inconsistent or insensitive manner;

- some parents have had to endure multiple funerals as organs or tissues were returned on several separate occasions;

- the scale of retention of organs was in many cases disproportionate and unnecessary for the underlying clinical condition or the focus of research activity.

17   It is an insufficient and inadequate explanation for the events to say that the law governing the practices was technically adhered to. In some places, there is clear evidence that custom and practice has departed from the legal framework. Even leaving this aside, parents and relatives are bound to say that within the law there was a better, more humane and more caring way in which those responsible could have operated the system. Improvements have been made, but many will see this as having been driven by crisis and occurring too late in the day to be of comfort to the majority who have suffered.

"Many of the parents also say if they were asked if organs could be used for research they would have consented."

Lynne Langley
Stolen Hearts Group
Speaking at the CMO's Summit on 11th January 2001

18   It is a tribute to those who have suffered in this way that they so clearly accept the benefits to medical science and the quality of health care that the study of organs and tissues after death can bring. If they had been asked, in the right way, they would have wanted their child's death to have helped someone else. Their sense of loss is heightened by the fact that much retained material was not used.

The practice in Bristol

- Tissues and organs had, over a long period of time, been systematically taken at or after post-mortem on babies and children who had died following paediatric cardiac surgery.

- The tissue and organs removed and retained were used for a variety of purposes including audit, medical education or research or had simply been stored.

- When coroners' post-mortems were carried out, parents were not told that the pathologist might take or retain tissue or organs, or the uses to which retained tissue and organs might be put. Consent was not sought.

- When hospital post-mortems were carried out, 'consent forms' were often signed but there was little information on what tissue or organs would be taken or the uses to which they might be put.

- The term 'tissue' was not defined. In particular it was not explained that this could include whole organs.

The practice at Alder Hey

- As in Bristol, tissues and organs had been systematically taken at post-mortems on babies or children who had died over a long period of time.

- Between 1988 and 1995, all organs were removed from all babies and children on whom post-mortems were conducted;

- Still-born babies and fetuses were also kept, or their organs and tissue retained.

- There is evidence that clinicians failed even to determine whether parents objected, let alone provide adequate information as a basis for a decision.

- The large majority of retained organs and tissue were not examined nor were they used for medical education or research purposes. They were simply stored against the possibility of being used in future research, which did not materialise.

- No choices were offered on methods of disposal of retained tissue and organs.

- Further samples of tissue were taken from organs before they were returned to families for subsequent burial.

- In some cases, families appear to have been pressurised into agreeing to a hospital post-mortem under threat of a coroner's post-mortem for which no consent is required.

- Consent to post-mortem, which was given, was exceeded or ignored where families had sought to limit the extent of the post-mortem examination (eg. to an existing operative incision, limited to specific organs or restricting the retention of organs or tissue).

- Families were misinformed about the organs and tissue retained after post-mortems on their babies or children.

- The term "tissue" was not explained. In particular, it was not made clear that this could include whole organs especially in small babies. Most parents who thought about it imagined that tissue meant small amounts of tissue for microscopic examination.

What are the problems with past and current practice?

19   The disturbing revelations from Bristol, Alder Hey and elsewhere highlight a number of areas where past and current practice is out of step with public expectations.

a) Consent Practice

The Human Tissue Act 1961 relies on establishing 'lack of objection' as the test to authorise the removal and retention of body parts. The wording of forms in common use throughout the NHS, as revealed by the census, reflects this rather than requiring 'consent' or agreement.

A signed form was used by 97% of Trusts to record lack of objection to post-mortem and 92% of Trusts used either the same or a separate form to obtain lack of objection to retention of organs and tissue. The fact that the Act requires the person authorising the removal of any body parts to 'have no reason to believe' that there is any objection, requires only that that person makes "such reasonable enquiry as may be practicable" without any further specification of what that might involve. In effect, relatives were asked to sign forms which were 'agreement that they did not object'. This is out of step with current thinking on the need for bereaved families to be given sufficient information in order to reach a decision and subject to any views that a deceased adult may have expressed, to be equal partners in the decision making process.

"From our perspective there has been a very large change in the extent to which the public wish to be informed and consulted, or perhaps it is a change in their ability to voice that need which has probably always been there, and we support that very much. We would accept that in many cases the profession has been slow to keep up with that big cultural change."

Professor Ian Booth
Royal College of Paediatrics and Child Health
Speaking at the CMO's Summit on 11th January 2001

Problems with 'consent' forms in current use

- recording 'lack of objection' rather than consent;
- lack of options for relatives to refuse or limit the post-mortem to express specific wishes about the retention of organs and tissue;
- 'tissue' not defined and usually no indication that it might cover the retention of whole organs;
- no choices for relatives on how retained tissue or organs were to be disposed of.

The report of the census of organs and tissues held by pathology services in England provides more detail (see www.doh.gov.uk/organcensus).

b) Provision of Information

Families have traditionally been given little information on the post-mortem examination itself or on tissue and organ retention, either to explain the practices or procedures or the potential longer term benefits for medical care for others of such procedures.

Families have not been made aware of the choices available to them in terms of limiting the extent of a hospital post-mortem, or the tissue or organs to be retained (if any) or the period for which they may be retained. Because coroners' post-mortems do not require the family's consent (or even 'lack of objection'), little information has been given to families on the procedures to be followed.

No information on the definition of tissue or organs is routinely provided. In particular, if 'tissue' is mentioned there is rarely, if ever any indication that this could cover whole organs. The Human Tissue Act 1961 itself provides no definition.

"The authority form to conduct a hospital post mortem was misleading. The word "tissue" implied to many parents a sliver or pinch of tissue to be examined under a microscope, it did not imply organs or, in some instances, whole body systems being removed and retained."

Lynne Langley
Stolen Hearts Group
Speaking at the CMO's Summit on 11th January 2001

c) Retention of organs and tissue without apparent consent

Organs and tissues have been retained following post-mortems without lack of objection having been established under the Human Tissue Act 1961. In the census, 16,000 organs were reported as retained (beyond the point necessary to establish the cause of death) following coroners' post-mortems between 1970 and 1999. This was despite the lack of a power for the coroner to direct or allow this or any authority for the pathologist to do so without the consent of relatives. The retention of tissue was even more common, with tissue having been retained from one-third of coroners' post-mortems over the period.

d) Poor Record Keeping

It became apparent at Alder Hey, when the hospital authorities started the process of returning organs and tissue to parents for further funerals, that there were serious deficiencies in the records:

- no proper record of retained organs or any audit trail of their taking and use;
- no record of the access granted to them for research purposes, so that there was no opportunity to inform parents of any research use made of their children's tissue or organs;
- lack of linkages between the Trust and the University's records so that new tissue and organ collections came to light for parents who had already had organs returned and held funerals.

In the process of conducting the census it has become apparent that these deficiencies are not restricted to Alder Hey. The figures given in the census are in many cases estimates. Full cataloguing will provide more accurate numbers of retained tissues and organs.

e) Disposal

It has been taken for granted by NHS authorities, and is in line with current law and guidance, that human tissue removed after surgery or removed at post-mortem and no longer required, should be incinerated as clinical waste. While the need for respect for, and sensitive disposal of, fetuses and stillborn babies has increasingly been recognised over the past decade, the same respect has not been accorded to organs and tissue, even those from babies and children who have died. This has come as a surprise and a shock to many. There is particular revulsion, for many, at the categorisation of part of a loved one as 'clinical waste' and strong objection to the concept of incineration as opposed to cremation.

f) Bereavement

Past and current practice has relied upon relatives being asked to sign a form to authorise post-mortems shortly after death – in some cases shortly after the news of the death has broken. At such a time, families need time to come to terms with their grief. Where a post-mortem is being suggested, families need to be provided with support and supplied with clear factual and unbiased information. At all times they need to be treated with dignity and respect.

"In accordance with those recommendations, we would like to see that relatives are given proper time to reflect on whether or not consent should be given. They should not be pressurised to sign anything on the spot and they should certainly be given the opportunity to discuss their decision with their religious advisors."

David Frei
Registrar of Beth Din
Speaking at the CMO's Summit on 11th January 2001

The Interim Guidance on Post-Mortem examination issued by the Department of Health last year required NHS Trusts to designate a named individual to provide this support and information to families of the deceased, whether a post-mortem is requested by a hospital doctor or the coroner. Many NHS Trusts now have such an individual, but further recognition of the importance of the role of a bereavement adviser and provision of standard professional training may be needed to ensure that all families requiring such support have access to it.

g) Religion and culture

It is clear from my discussions with different religious leaders and from evidence given to the National Summit that the support available is not always as aware of, or sensitive to, the needs of different cultures and religions around the time of death as it should be. It is important that the clinical team as a whole, in addition to the bereavement adviser, is aware of these needs, for example the importance in the Jewish and Muslim religions of burying the body intact, wherever possible, and as soon as possible.

"We believe that it is very important that all staff coming into contact with bereaved parents and their families have an awareness of the cultural background within which the individuals operate. A significant number of individuals would find the process of histological or post-mortem examination abhorrent to them and we believe that this wish, expect where it is over-ridden by the need for a coroner's inquest, should always be respected."

Louise Silverton
The Royal College of Midwives

Training for all health professionals in how to support bereaved relatives at the time of death needs to be sensitive to cultural and religious requirements. Standard literature needs to be available in different languages, geared to the stance of the wide range of different cultures in this country, and the team dealing with the family needs to be able to communicate with them in their own language. Perhaps most importantly, NHS Trusts need to work in partnership with the community they serve, to develop working arrangements for providing support around the death of a loved one which take full account of different cultural and religious beliefs.

Conclusions

20   Past and current practice as described above has a number of significant weaknesses. There has been:

- a lack of respect for the dead and for the feelings of bereaved relatives in the arrangements for taking and disposing of organs and tissues following post-mortem examination;

- inadequate provision of clear information about what the post-mortem examination entails, both when the post-mortem is requested by the coroner and when requested by the hospital doctor, which has prevented families making informed decisions;

- little consultation with families on the future use of any tissue and organs they agree to being retained;

- poor and inappropriate bereavement support in many NHS Trusts;

- witting or unwitting breaches of the Human Tissue Act 1961, particularly in respect of retaining tissues and organs beyond the time necessary to establish the cause of death following coroners' post-mortems;

- failure to involve families as equal partners in the process of making decisions about their loved one who has died;

- no systematic attempt to explain the potential benefits of medical research on organs and tissue retained at post-mortem. All the indications are that, approached in the proper way, with honesty and provision of the information families want, that many would agree to the retention of organs and tissue for research;

- disposal of human organs, tissue and body parts following post-mortem as clinical waste which many people find unacceptable. Choice and respect for the families' wishes about disposing of retained organs and tissues have been largely absent, except where stillborn babies and fetuses are concerned.

4

Related issues

Previous chapters have considered the legal framework underpinning the practice of taking and retaining organs from post-mortem and deficiencies in current practice. This chapter considers a number of related issues which need to be taken into account in a new and comprehensive system.

The Coroners System

1   The provisions of the coroners legislation reflect the fact that the coroner's main purpose is to investigate suspicious or unexpected deaths. It is clear why there is no provision for consent from relatives in the most extreme cases. However, many of the cases which fall to be referred to the coroner, such as death during recovery from an operation, or sudden death where a person has not been attended by their general practitioner for 14 days are of a different nature.

2   The current system raises a number of concerns:

- families are not provided with information on the process nor do they regularly receive feedback of the results of the post-mortem: indeed this is rarely provided to treating clinicians;

- coroners' post-mortems, whose only purpose is to establish cause of death for death certification, do not as currently carried out provide sufficient information for clinicians to enable them to make improvements in standards of care or for the performance of individual clinicians or units to be assessed and audited;

- a pathologist carrying out a post-mortem examination on behalf of the coroner can limit his or her examination solely to establishing the cause of death;

- the decision whether or not to refer to a coroner may be influenced by the referring clinician under whose care the patient may have died.

3   This has led to concerns about the overall quality of coroners' post-mortems. They are not undertaken to a common standard, they need not conform to best practice guidelines for post-mortem examination and they may not be thorough enough to serve as an audit of the person's care. There is anecdotal evidence that some coroners are limiting the examination further by asking that organs are not removed for examination, even in situations where the pathologist might deem it necessary for a proper examination.

4   It is important that the public receive value for the services carried out. About £12 million is paid out to pathologists in fees for coroners' post-mortems. A total of approximately £35 million is paid each year by relatives for medical certificates for cremation.

5   A major review of the coroners system would have significant advantages. It could consider ways of reconciling the different functions: establishing the cause of death in unexpected or suspicious circumstances and providing information to families, clinicians and the health service more generally, not only on cause of death, but on clinical performance, audit and standards.

6   Such a review could include consideration of a 'medical examiner' system. A medical examiner could:

- provide an independent expert review of the circumstances of death and provide feedback to relatives and the registrar of deaths on the cause of death and to clinicians and NHS management on the cause of death and standards of practice;

"We believe that it is the duty and responsibility of the coroner's office to explain the needs for post mortem examination to relatives. There appears to be great variability in the skill with which this is done and, indeed, whether it is done at all."

Patricia Wilkie
Patients' Liaison Group
Royal College of Pathologists
Speaking at the CMO's Summit on 11th January 2001

- operate with informed consent from families and in accordance with their expressed wishes;

- authorise retention of tissue and organs following post-mortem in accordance with the family's wishes or arrange respectful disposal, again in accordance with the family's wishes;

- inspect registers of deaths held by health authorities;

- liaise with funeral directors, registrars, police, local hospital and primary care clinical governance leads.

Death Certification

7   The Home Office is currently conducting a review of death certification introduced in response to the conviction of Dr Harold Shipman. This aims to review the current system of registration of deaths and make recommendations for improvements. The process of death registration in England and Wales is complex and is governed by laws and regulations accumulated over more than a century and a half. Information gathered through the death certification process is used for public health planning and evaluation, clinical research, resource allocation and a variety of other purposes. As we have seen, coroners investigate about a quarter of all deaths, but the system is not currently designed to provide reliable, uniform, good quality information on deaths from diseases for public health purposes, for medical research or for improving standards of care.

8   The most radical option proposed in the Home Office review proposes the introduction of a medical examiner who would confirm the cause of death (see above), determine whether there needed to be an inquest, authorise the disposal of the body and provide an overview of deaths in the area. This has clear links to the elements of a review of the coroners system outlined above.

9   The Home Office review of death certification should be linked to a wider review of the coroners system to provide a fundamental re-evaluation of the approach to establishing and recording the cause of death and providing feedback to families, clinicians and NHS management.

Importation of Body Parts

10   Neither the Anatomy Act 1984 nor the Human Tissue Act 1961 covers the importation of limbs or body parts. As surgery and training in new surgical techniques is not permitted under the Anatomy Act, a small number of centres in recent years have arranged for the importation of frozen limbs from abroad. The purposes for which these imports have been made include:

- demonstration of specialised surgical anatomy and surgical techniques to surgeons and therapists in training;

- to permit established surgeons to practise microsurgical and new and complex techniques on limbs where accidental damage during operative surgery could harm patients;

- to explore biomechanical aspects of inserting new joint replacements in limbs.

11   Imports of frozen limbs are known to have been received by a small number of hospitals, who have reported taking up to 100 limbs, mainly from the United States of America. It is not known whether all hospitals involved in such importations have been identified.

12   While limbs donated under the Human Tissue Act could be used for the purposes for which limbs have been imported, it appears that surgeons have been reluctant to seek consent from relatives in this country.

13   As importation of body parts is not controlled by any statutory regime, there is a further Public Health consideration arising from the import of frozen human body parts. In the absence of any regulatory system it is currently left to the individual or organisation importing human body parts to decide for themselves on safety questions. Frozen limbs and organs have the potential to transmit viral and other infections and may not meet the safety standards that apply in this country to prevent transmission of infection.

14   The ethical and legal requirements in countries from which frozen limbs are obtained may also be different from this country. Those who import frozen limbs or other body parts can only rely on the documentation provided that the body part has been lawfully and ethically obtained.

15   Any comprehensive review of the law on human tissue should encompass controls on the importation of body parts from abroad. While this should not necessarily be banned, controls will be needed to ensure that imported limbs have been obtained ethically, removed safely and that they have been subjected to appropriate screening to rule out the risk of infection.

Commercial Use of Human Tissue

16   Human tissue is used in the production of commercial cell lines which support pharmaceutical and biomedical research in both universities and private industry. Such uses include the development of vaccines. They are not sold to commercial companies although a 'handling fee' may be paid to NHS Trusts. It is doubtful whether consent has been sought for

such use and many people have concerns about profit being made from human tissue and body parts. The growing potential of DNA analysis of human tissue to unlock the key to a wide range of diseases means that there needs to be absolute clarity about the intended uses of tissue when consent is sought. The question of the commercial use of tissue should be included in any wider review of the law in this area.

Tissue Banks

17   It was estimated in 1994 that some 10,000 procedures in the NHS involve a human tissue transplant. Tissue is processed and stored in a range of 'banks'. Recent estimates indicate that there are around 80 formal tissue banks in the UK. The majority of them are fairly large and are under the auspices of the British Association of Tissue Banks or the UK National Blood Transfusion Service. Anecdotal evidence suggests that many 'informal' tissue banks are also operating within the NHS.

18   Department of Health guidance has been issued on the basic requirements of donor screening, but there has been no national system to monitor compliance, to ensure that tissue can be traced from donor to recipient, or to ensure that storage standards are satisfactory.

19   Following consultation, a non-statutory regulatory UK wide system is now being established for human tissue banks to provide assurances on the safety and quality of human tissue used therapeutically.

20   Organisations providing human tissue for therapeutic purposes will need to apply for accreditation. They must also function ethically, obtaining proper consent. The sale of human organs and tissue is prohibited. Organisations providing human tissue for therapeutic purposes will be permitted to recover the costs of supplying the tissue but not to make a profit. NHS Chief Executives will be required only to use tissue from an accredited source.

21   There are currently no restrictions on the import of human tissue to the UK. Safety standards may vary depending on its source. Therefore it is important to ensure that imported tissue meets the same safety standards as tissue from within the UK. Under the non-statutory regime, the individual or organisation importing human tissue must reassure themselves that the tissue meets the requirements of standards of tissue banking in the UK. However, at present, these standards do not have the force of law.

5 Conclusions and Recommendations

This chapter presents the overall conclusions drawn from my consideration of this complex subject and recommendations on the way forward.

1   The discovery by parents in Bristol, Liverpool and other cities that large numbers of children's organs and tissues had been kept after post-mortem examination without their knowledge or permission has caused a public outcry. This has focused attention on major weaknesses in the way this area of practice has operated and been governed over many years.

2   These events have been the subject of two major inquiries and reports – the interim report of the Bristol Royal Infirmary Inquiry and the Royal Liverpool Children's NHS Trust (Alder Hey) Inquiry Report. The inquiries have led to the establishment of a number of groups representing parents who have campaigned to draw their experience to the attention of the public and those in positions of authority as well as making many valuable proposals for change.

> *"there must be an immediate change in the law. The rules governing hospital and coroners' post mortems must be the same. Doctors must be obliged to seek fully informed consent from families for the examination of the relative's body and the retention of every item of material. Contravention must lead to disciplinary action ...*
>
> *Cultural change: education of the profession about pathology, in communicating with the bereaved, education of the public about practices and procedures relating to pathology and a new spirit of openness and clarity between the medical profession and the public, which NACOR are trying to do at present."*
>
> Michaela Willis
> NACOR
> Speaking at the CMO's Summit on 11th January 2001

3   With the benefit of hindsight the situation in Bristol, Liverpool and other hospitals was out of step with public expectations. Considerable holdings of organs, body parts, tissues and fetuses had been accumulating over many decades. The law governing this practice is unclear, ambiguous and ageing. The law was, in any event poorly understood and, as a result not applied well. Custom and practice developed within this framework of law which relied too heavily on a traditional and rather paternalistic attitude in which the benefit of teaching and research were seen as self-evident truths and the wishes and feelings of individual parents and families were not sufficiently recognised.

4   This report has analysed the issues underlying the controversy. It draws on the experience of families caught up in these events; on information provided by the two inquiries; on

information from a census of NHS pathology services in England carried out in 2000; on the evidence given to a National Summit on 11 January 2001; and on the views and ideas of a wide range of individuals and organisations.

5 Around 105,000 organs, body parts, stillbirths and fetuses were reported as being held in pathology departments and medical schools in England at the end of 1999. About half had been accumulated over the last thirty years, whilst the remainder dated from pre-1970 and were part of historical collections or archives. Other countries, including the United States of America, maintain large repositories of human tissue and organs for research, treatment and educational purposes.

6 In England, the retention of organs and tissues after death are permitted in two main circumstances:

- after a post-mortem examination ordered by a coroner. The retention is only permissible for the time necessary to establish the cause of death and not for research or teaching;

- after a hospital post-mortem carried out under the auspices of the Human Tissue Act 1961 where long term retention for teaching or research can take place if it is established that relatives 'do not object' (or that the deceased before death 'did not object').

7 Past practice in England, which has resulted in the stored organs and tissues, has operated within the current legal framework, as supplemented by NHS and professional guidance. At times it appears to have ignored or deviated from the law (for example long term retention of tissue or organs occurred after coroners post-mortem examination when this does not appear to be permitted by the law). At Alder Hey Hospital, the inquiry identified more flagrant abuses of the law. On the whole, whilst conforming to the letter of the law, practice has fallen well short of a sensitive and modern system of seeking and obtaining consent to hospital post-mortem or to the longer term retention of tissue and organs for medical education, teaching or research.

8 This has allowed a system to become established which has failed to engage families as partners in the decisions about their child's body after death.

> *"When a child died that child is still the parents' child – not a specimen, not a cause, not an unfortunate casualty of a failed procedure, but someone's baby, someone's child. In life the parent is responsible for every aspect of a child's well-being. In death that responsibility should not be taken away."*
>
> Stephen Parker
> Bristol Heart Children's Action Group
> Speaking at the CMO's Summit on 11th January 2001

9 This has undermined the strong bedrock of support for advancing medical science and contributing to higher standards of care which undoubtedly exists amongst the public of this country. Even families caught up in the worst of the recent events have said that they would have been willing to donate their loved one's organ or tissue to help others had they been asked properly.

10 The overwhelming conclusion of the majority of commentators is that the system and the law in this area must be changed so that proper involvement of families can enable their support to be gained in the pursuit of the conquest of disease and excellence in standards of health care.

11   Poor cataloguing and recording of retained tissue and organs, both in hospitals and in University research collections, has been highlighted by events at Alder Hey. The consequential distress from the second, third and fourth funerals that some families have faced must not be repeated for other families. The lack of accurate records has also meant that there has been no feedback to families on any research on their child's organs, which may have provided some degree of comfort. Against this, however, it is important to recognise that in many research collections on which legitimate research has been undertaken it may not always be possible to tie remaining samples to individuals.

12   The practice of disposing of tissue and organs, after post-mortem or where no longer required for research use, as clinical waste is shocking to many people. This is not seen as according due respect to the dead or the feelings of bereaved families. More respectful disposal through cremation or burial should be available for those who want it.

13   Perhaps as a result of the difficulty that our society has with addressing the question of death, the necessary support for the bereaved has largely, until recently, been lacking in our hospitals. Silence, embarrassment and half truths have substituted for openness, provision of information, sensitivity and dialogue.

14   My recommendations are underpinned by a set of guiding principles set out below:

Guiding principles

- Respect: treating the person who has died and their families with dignity and respect.

- Understanding: realising that to many parents and families their love and feelings of responsibility for the person who has died are as strong as they were in life.

- Informed consent: ensuring that permission is sought and given on the basis that a person is exercising fully informed choice; consent is a process not a 'one off' event.

- Time and space: recognising that a family member may need time to consider whether to agree to a post-mortem examination and to consider donation of tissue and organs and will not wish to feel under pressure to agree in the moments after death.

- Skill and sensitivity: NHS staff must be sensitive to the needs of the relatives of someone who has died and sufficient staff skilled in bereavement counselling must be available.

- Information: much better information is required, both generally by the public and specifically for relatives who are recently bereaved, about post-mortems and the use of tissue after death. Relatives may also require information about the progress of research involving donated material.

- Cultural competence: attitudes to post-mortem examination, burial, and the use of organs and tissues after death differ greatly between different religions and cultural groups; health professionals need to be aware of these factors and respond to them with sensitivity.

- A gift relationship: the emphasis in all present legislation and guidance is on 'taking' and 'retaining'. The balance should be shifted to 'donation', so that tissue or organs are given as a gift to help others and recognised as deserving of gratitude to those making donations.

15   Examination of the professional practices and law which have given rise to organ and tissue retention raises issues for the coroners system and whether it meets modern day needs; the system of death certification; and the broader issues of the controls that are needed on taking, storing and using tissue and organs from both the living and the dead.

16   Special attention will need to be given to older collections, archives and repositories of organs and tissues which using new techniques of scientific analysis may contain medical information of international importance.

Recommendations

17   The framing of these recommendations has drawn heavily on the well-informed recommendations in the Bristol Interim Inquiry Report and also the conclusions and insights provided by the Alder Hey Inquiry Report. In the light of my analysis of the problems with the current system and the principles set out earlier, the following recommendations are made:

Recommendation 1: **As an immediate measure, the Human Tissue Act 1961 should be amended to clarify that consent must be sought from those with parental responsibility for the retention of tissue or organs from post-mortems on children beyond the time necessary to establish the cause of death. A penalty for non-compliance with the provisions of the Human Tissue Act 1961 should be introduced.**

The Human Tissue Act 1961 requires a hospital to satisfy itself that relatives have no objection to the removal of any part of the body for purposes of medical education and research. However, that Act contains no penalties for breach of its provisions. This would be rectified if this recommendation is implemented. There has been a lack of clarity over the circumstances in which tissue and organs may be retained after a coroner's post-mortem (for which no consent is required).

The proposal to limit the amendment to the retention of tissue and organs from children recognises the immense distress that such retentions without the parents' knowledge and consent have caused. It will also be more straightforward to implement than provisions relating to adults where it would be necessary to define the categories of persons entitled to give consent.

Recommendation 2: **the Coroners Rules 1984 should be amended to clarify that the pathologist has no independent right to retain, use or dispose of human material once the Coroner's post-mortem is concluded, except on the authority of the Coroner in, for example, criminal cases, or with the consent of parents.**

The ambiguity which is contained within Rule 9 of the Coroners Rules has clearly led to the retention of tissues and organs for longer than necessary to establish the cause of death and for purposes other than those covered by coroners' statutory powers. This is clear from the census and from the two Inquiry Reports and is specifically drawn attention to in the recommendations of the Bristol Interim Inquiry Report. Given that relatives do not have a choice in whether a coroners' post-mortem is carried out, an early change to the law is required to clarify that there should be no such retention under coroners legislation. Separate consent would need to be sought under the amended Human Tissue Act 1961 (see Recommendation 1 above).

Recommendation 3: **A Code of Practice, supported by Directions from the Secretary of State for Health under the National Health Service Act 1977, should be introduced as soon as possible, to set out the required standards of practice in communications with families about both hospital and coroners' post-mortems.**

A Code of Practice would support the immediate changes to the law outlined in Recommendation 1 and would set out good practice on decision-making and communication on post-mortems and retention of organs and tissue after post-mortem for both children and adults.

It would cover the standards required for communication on both hospital and coroners' post-mortems, including for example:

- the information to be given to families following post-mortem;

- the need for consent to hospital post-mortems, who should seek that consent and who can give it;

- the need for consent to the retention of tissues and organs beyond the time necessary to establish the cause of death;

- details of the tissue and organs to be retained, the uses to which they might be put, and the agreed length of time for retention;

- the opportunity for parents/families to refuse or to restrict the use of their relative's tissue or organs;

- providing the family with a permanent record of the discussion and agreement reached and including a copy in the patient record;

- maintaining proper documentation of all tissues and organs retained so that at any time the location and use of these is recorded. This record should also include details of when and how disposal is undertaken;

- respectful disposal of tissue and organs in accordance with any wishes expressed by families.

The Code of Practice could be supported in the NHS by Directions from the Secretary of State for Health under the National Health Service Act 1977, and should be brought to the attention of coroners by the Home Office and Coroners' Society. Breach of the provisions of the Code should be a disciplinary offence within the NHS.

Recommendation 4: **A standardised consent form should be provided for use throughout the NHS to obtain consent to hospital post-mortems and, separately, to the retention of tissue and organs following post-mortem.**

The census of organ and tissue retention practice indicated that a standardised form to record 'lack of objection' to a hospital post-mortem or retention of 'tissue' has been in use in many hospitals, apparently for many years. More recently, individual NHS Trusts have sought to develop improvements in their forms to offer more explanation and opportunities for families to express choices. However, few of the examples provided with the returns to the census are without problems. A standardised form should therefore be developed. Amongst its key features as proposed by the Bristol Interim Inquiry Report should be:

- clear definitions of 'tissue'; 'organs', and 'blocks';

- options for refusing or placing limitations on the hospital post-mortem; eg limiting examination to particular organs;

- options for refusing or limiting the organs or tissue to be retained or the uses to which they might be put;

- options for limiting the time for which organs or tissue might be retained;

- options for the subsequent disposal of retained tissue and organs;

- requiring the form to be witnessed;

- a copy of the consent form to be provided to the family and included in the patient record.

The outline new consent form proposed by the Alder Hey Inquiry – reproduced in the Inquiry report – provides a starting point and should be developed by the Department of Health in consultation with parent and other patient groups and professional bodies.

Recommendation 5: **An independent Commission should be established to oversee the proper return of retained organs and tissues to families who request it and to address the question of historical and archived collections obtained from post-mortem examinations. The role of HM Inspector of Anatomy should be broadened to assist with these tasks.**

The census has indicated that there are significant holdings of tissue, organs, stillbirths and fetuses retained from 1970 onwards and significant holdings in archive and museum collections dating from before 1970. It is important to ensure that these are dealt with sensitively and effectively by the NHS and Universities. The new Commission would:

- ensure that there are accurate records and catalogues before any returns to families are made (to avoid multiple funerals);

- ensure that NHS Trusts and Universities work together to provide a complete record of retentions identifiable to a particular family;

- ensure that families are involved in agreeing with NHS Trusts procedures for dignified return or disposal;

- provide an advocacy service for families experiencing difficulties obtaining information from their local NHS Trust;

- provide advice (after consultation) to the Government and to NHS Trusts and Universities on the return, retention, further use or disposal of archive and museum collections, some of which are of international medical importance.

The particular issues for the return of organs from research collections, some of which may have been used as part of legitimate research projects, will also need to be addressed by the Commission.

The post of HM Inspector of Anatomy has ensured the rigorous regulation of donation and use of a dead body for anatomical teaching in medical schools. The Inspector's expertise should be used by the new Commission.

Recommendation 6: As soon as possible, there should be a more fundamental and broader revision of the law, encompassing the taking, storage and use of human tissue from the living and the dead and introducing an independent system of regulatory control. To be comprehensive this should encompass aspects of coroners' practice. It should shift the emphasis from 'retention' to 'donation' to signal a new relationship with the public and bereaved families.

There would need to be widespread consultation on detailed proposals for such a major revision of the law (which would need to be developed in consultation between the Department of Health, the Home Office and the Lord Chancellor's Department).

The purpose of the new legislation would be to establish a clear and comprehensive regime governing the donation and all uses of human tissue, for which there is an existing model under the Anatomy Act 1984. This could:

- provide a statutory basis for regulating all aspects of obtaining, storage, use and disposal of all tissue and organs;

- set out a detailed exposition of who could give consent to taking and using tissue and organs in life and after death, for therapeutic purposes, for research and for educational purposes;

- introduce a regulatory body with responsibility for providing guidance on compliance with the law; inspecting the storage of tissues and organs; regulating use; and providing annual returns on tissue and organs retained and the uses to which they are put.

This fundamental review should incorporate a review of the Anatomy Act 1984 to ensure that the fundamental principles and regulatory regime of that Act apply to all retentions of human tissues.

The inter-relationship between the Coroners system, death certification and any changes proposed need to be considered as part of the review.

Recommendation 7: Formal controls should be introduced on the import and export of body parts.

The comprehensive review of the law recommended at Recommendation 6 should encompass consideration of the need for a system of controls on the importation of body parts. This should include provisions to ensure that such body parts have been obtained ethically, that the appropriate consents have been obtained, and that they have been subject to specified screening to rule out the risk of infection.

Pending the fundamental review of the law proposed in recommendation 6 a Code of Practice should be introduced to require that proper records are maintained by those arranging such imports. The records should include details of the reason for importation, the source, provenance, actual use and disposal of all human body parts brought into the country for teaching, education, research or other purposes. Details of the individual or organisation responsible for the importation should be maintained. The Code of Practice should require a similar record to be kept of all body parts, and organs, exported from this country.

Recommendation 8: The ultimate disposal of retained tissues, organs, body parts, stillbirths and fetuses should be in accordance with any expressed wishes of the individual or his or her family.

The practice of incinerating retained tissues, organs and body parts as clinical waste should be reviewed in association with crematoria authorities and funeral directors as well as the public, with the aim of offering cremation or burial where this is a family's preferred option. In the case of an adult, disposal should be in accordance with any expressed wishes of the deceased or the views of the family or those closest to the deceased. In the case of a child, the parent's views should be sought and respected.

The Cremation (Amendment) Regulations 2000 allow for the cremation of tissue and organs retained after post-mortem where the body has previously been buried. These provisions should be extended to stillbirths and to body parts retained under the Anatomy Act 1984.

Provisions relating to the cremation or burial of pre-viable fetuses and subsequently for any tissues retained need clarification. Families should be invited to express their wishes on disposal and those wishes should be respected.

Recommendation 9: **Time limits should be specified for the retention of tissue blocks and slides retained after post-mortem.**

Tissue blocks and slides taken at post-mortem have traditionally been retained as part of the medical record and kept more or less indefinitely. There is considerable value in this retention for follow-up investigations on the illness of the deceased, diagnosis of other family members in the case of genetic disorders and long term investigation of disease and treatment. However, wholesale retention on a permanent basis does not appear to be justified. Moreover, some families have objected to the retention of blocks of tissues which are substantial parts of organs. The comprehensive review of the law recommended at Recommendation 6 should include consideration of setting time limits for the retention of blocks and slides, taking account of the scientific and legal needs for such retention, and public views. In the short term the Commission proposed at Recommendation 5 should provide advice to NHS Trusts.

Recommendation 10: **The Coroners' system as it relates to hospital deaths and deaths under the care of a general practitioner should be reviewed and the concept of introducing a 'medical examiner' system should be explored.**

Recommendation 11: **The feasibility of establishing a new system of death certification involving a medical examiner should be explored.**

The function of the Coroners' system of establishing the cause of death in unexpected or suspicious circumstances, does not sit easily with currently identified needs to provide information to families, clinicians and the health services on both cause of death and on clinical performance.

Consideration should be given to the introduction of a 'medical examiner' system, in which the medical examiner would provide an independent expert review of the cause of death; provide feedback to the relatives of the deceased on the cause of death; operate with informed consent from families and authorise retention of tissue and organs at post-mortem, where they agreed, for future study or for educational purposes.

The Home Office's consultation on death certification proposes, as its most radical option, the introduction of a medical referee or medical examiner who would take over some of the existing functions of the Registrar of Births and Deaths, the second doctor certifying death if the patient is to be cremated, and, to some extent the coroner.

The medical examiner would:

- confirm the cause of deaths notified by the certifying doctor;
- exercise the present powers of the coroner to determine whether the death needed to be subject to an inquest;
- authorise disposal of the body;
- monitor and provide an overview of deaths in the health authority area.

The detail of a possible "medical examiner" system would need to be fully reviewed and the resulting recommendations would need to be subject to full public consultation but it could also help to address some of the issues raised by the Harold Shipman case.

Recommendation 12: All NHS Trusts should provide support and advice to families at the time of bereavement.

This support should include the services of a bereavement adviser who can help families in the difficult period following death or, where the situation allows, to offer support through the dying process. Their role should be to:-

- provide information on the circumstances of death, and encouraging dialogue with the treating clinician;
- be sensitive and responsive to different religious and cultural beliefs;
- assist any family wishing to donate organs or tissue (or to carry out wishes of the deceased to do so), by making contact with the transplant co-ordination service or other appropriate arrangements;
- provide a full explanation of the reasons for post-mortem examination, including therapeutic uses, medical education and research;
- explain the need for consent to carry out a hospital post-mortem and for consent to retaining organs following either a coroner's or hospital post-mortem;
- provide practical assistance to families on all the official procedures which need to be undertaken after a death.

Training will be needed for bereavement advisers to understand the different views of death in different cultures; to understand the post-mortem procedures and issues of consent; and in the psychological component of sensitive and respectful communication.

Recommendation 13: Research using donated tissue and organs taken at post-mortem can provide valuable information on disease, treatments and standards of care. It should be promoted where families have given informed consent to tissue or organs from their deceased relative being used in that way. There should be feedback to families on the research use of donated tissue or organs where requested. For tissue and organs donated for teaching, families should be invited to prepare a 'life book' on the child (or adult) who has died which would be shown to students in conjunction with the use of the tissue or organ for teaching.

There are serious concerns that the great value of medical research and education using tissue and organs taken at post-mortem will be lost, as families will be reluctant to give their consent. Some families will indeed refuse such consent. This is their right now, as it has been in the past. However many of the families affected by the tragedies in Bristol and at Alder Hey have indicated that they would have consented if the purposes of retention had been explained and they had been asked.

In the short-term, the Code of Practice recommended at Recommendation 3 will set out the standards of practice in obtaining consent for research use. It will also require accurate record keeping and links to patient records, which will enable families to be given information on any research project for which their relative's tissue and organs have been used, if they wish. These aspects should be included in the comprehensive review of the law proposed at Recommendation 6.

The 'life book', which might include photographs of the child or any information which the parents wanted to provide, would help to ensure that the value of the donation could not be forgotten, and would encourage an attitude of respect and awareness of the fundamental human nature of the tissues and organs being used for teaching and avoid them becoming dehumanised objects.

Recommendation 14: **There should be a programme of public education to ensure that there is general understanding of what is involved in the post-mortem process and its value to maintaining standards of patient care and medical science.**

Provision of information will set a climate of general understanding of what a post-mortem involves. Families faced with decisions about a loved one who has recently died will not then be confronted with the details for the first time in traumatic circumstances.

Such information might be provided through schools, general information leaflets, more open discussion of the issues in the media and through the proposed new patients' advocacy services in Trusts.

Recommendation 15: **There should be a programme of education and training for all health professionals on the meaning of the law and appropriate standards of practice.**

The Code of Practice proposed at Recommendation 3 will set out appropriate standards of practice for all NHS staff in obtaining consent to hospital post-mortem and subsequent retention and use of tissue and organs. This should be supported by updated guidance from professional bodies where necessary.

There is increasing recognition that communication skills should be incorporated in training programmes for all health professionals and this should continue. In addition, there needs to be a comprehensive programme of training to assist the whole clinical team, and bereavement advisers, to help support families at this difficult time.

Recommendation 16: **Procedures should be established (after public consultation) to provide for obtaining appropriate consent for research using stored human tissue.**

It is becoming apparent that new genetics techniques and other scientific developments will open up the opportunity for benefits to patients to come from the study of tissue or organs which are already in store. The prospect of donated organs or tissue being used for multiple

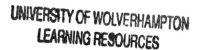

research purposes over many years is a complex issue where proper consultation is required before procedures are established. This work should build on the consultations already undertaken by the Medical Research Council.

Recommendation 17: **Research should be commissioned into less invasive forms of post-mortem examination.**

Proposals have been made that the use of magnetic resonance imaging and other scanning techniques could provide the benefits of post-mortem examination without the need for dissection of the body and the removal of organs. This would have particular advantages for some religious communities. The position is not clear and research should be commissioned to establish whether less invasive forms of post-mortem examination could be developed which would nevertheless provide a similar standard of information.

Annex: List of organisations and individuals invited to meet CMO/contribute to CMO's investigation

Professional Organisations:

Royal College of Pathologists

British Medical Association Medical Ethics Committee

Royal College of Nursing

United Kingdom Central Council for Nursing, Midwifery and Health Visiting

Coroners' Society for England and Wales

Confidential Enquiry into Stillbirths and Deaths in Infants

Religious and Ethnic Organisations:

Aga Khan Health Board

Al-Hasaniya Moroccan Women's Centre

Association of Community Interpreters and Translators, Advocates & Linkworkers

Association of Guyanese Nurses and Allied Professionals

Bishops' Conference Secretariat for England and Wales

Cancer Black Care

Central Mosque

Chief Rabbi's Office

Chinese Healthy Living Centre

Churches Commission for Racial Justice

Church of England Board of Responsibility

Confederation of African Organisations

Confederation of Indian Organisations

Council of British Pakistanis

East London Chinese Community Centre

Guild of Catholic Doctors

Hospital Chaplaincies Council

Institute for Jewish Policy Research

London Sickle Cell Trust

Mann Weaver

Mauritian Islamic Welfare Association

Mushkil Asaan

Muslim Council of Britain

N Films

National Council of Hindu Temples (UK)

Network of Sikh Organisations

New North London Masatori Synagogue

Rabbi Julia Neuberger

Reform Synagogues of Great Britain

Sangam Association of Asian Women

Swaminarayan Hindu Mission

The Refugee Council

The Synod

UK Action Committee on Islamic Affairs

Union of Liberal and Progressive Synagogues

West Indian Standing Conference

1990 Trust

Patients' representative groups

National Committee on Organ Retention (NACOR)

Patients Association

Patient Concern

PITY II

The Royal College of Pathologists Patients Liaison Committee